Strong is New Skinny:

Strength Training for Women, Exercise Manual for Stronger, Sexier and Curvier Body

Legal & Disclaimer

The information contained in this book and its contents is not designed to replace or take the place of any form of medical or professional advice; and is not meant to replace the need for independent medical, financial, legal or other professional advice or services, as may be required. The content and information in this book has been provided for educational and entertainment purposes only.

The content and information contained in this book has been compiled from sources deemed reliable, and it is accurate to the best of the Author's knowledge, information and belief. However, the Author cannot guarantee its accuracy and validity and cannot be held liable for any errors and/or omissions. Further, changes are periodically made to this book as and when needed. Where appropriate and/or necessary, you must consult a professional (including but not limited to your doctor, attorney, financial advisor or such other professional advisor) before using any of the suggested remedies, techniques, or information in this book.

Upon using the contents and information contained in this book, you agree to hold harmless the Author from and against any damages, costs, and expenses, including any legal fees potentially resulting from the application of any of the information provided by this book. This disclaimer applies to any loss, damages or injury caused by the use and application, whether directly or indirectly, of any advice or information presented, whether for breach of contract, tort, negligence, personal injury, criminal intent, or under any other cause of action.

You agree to accept all risks of using the information presented inside this book.

You agree that by continuing to read this book, where appropriate and/or necessary, you shall consult a professional (including but not limited to your doctor, attorney, or financial advisor or such other advisor as needed) before using any of the suggested remedies, techniques, or information in this book.

Table of Contents

Introduction

Strength training is an easy way for women to stay in shape while ensuring the continued bodily strength to live your life without restrictions. Another positive aspect of strength training is that you will avoid many problems and illnesses that are related to a sedentary lifestyle.

As you might already know, the older you become, the less active you tend to be, which causes muscles to lose their strength. However, by incorporating strength training, you will have an advantage, as it will help you to maintain a strong, lean and sculpted body for your entire life.

There is nothing to lose in taking up strength training but so much to win and there is no better workout for women as the benefits are countless.

Chapter 1: Benefits of Strength Training

Most people I know who have chosen to take up strength training, do so because they want to improve their physical appearance. When men take up strength training, they do develop substantial muscles. However, for women this isn't the case as the levels of testosterone in their bodies is substantially less. Through the right form of strength training, a woman can develop a much firmer (toned) physique. Plus over time they will start to see that they become much stronger.

However, one thing you should be aware of before you begin your strength training regime, which is something I was unaware of when I began mine, is that your genetic makeup will dictate the extent to which your body responds to the exercises you are doing.

But having said that, although you may not end up with a physique like Arnold Schwarzenegger or the likes of Jessica Ennis, you will soon reap the benefits of doing this form of training. Below we'll take a look at some of the main benefits:

As muscle mass increases over time so will your body's "Basal Metabolic Rate." In turn, you will start to notice that you lose fat more easily, plus keeping the fat off becomes a lot easier as well. Certainly, if you are someone who has tried various diets without any real success, then of course including strength training into your diet and fitness regime will prove extremely beneficial.

Furthermore, if you perform a very intense workout, you'll discover this helps to keep your metabolic rate elevated for many hours after you have completed your workout. This again will help you to lose fat more effectively and more quickly.

As your muscles become stronger, your posture will improve and in turn will provide your joints with much more support. This will then reduce the risk of you getting injured when carrying out other everyday activities.

As we get older, we lose some muscle tissue. Strength training can be a great way to counteract this. It can also be a great way to fight the signs of aging.

You don't have to take my word for it. If you search online, you'll find there are numerous reports available regarding studies that have been carried out which confirm this. In fact, the studies have included looking at people in their 80's and 90's who use strength training as part of their fitness regime.

Strength training plays a very important role in the rehabilitation of people who suffer from certain disabilities or following certain forms of surgery. By regularly performing certain strength training exercises, these people have found that strengthening of the muscles has helped them to recover from their illness much more quickly and effectively.

All athletes will include some form of strength training in their fitness regime as it helps to improve their performance. Today competitors, in a variety of different sports, will use strength-training routines that specifically relate to the sport that they are involved in.

This benefit relates to "all" exercises, not just strength training. Exercise helps to improve someone's mood as well as help alleviate any feelings of depression you may be having. The reason for this is that, through strength training, your body will begin to produce large amounts of chemicals in the body known as dopamine, serotonin, and norepinephrine which are all known for their mood enhancing qualities.

When a woman wants to tone her muscles, lose fat, or get her body firm. She will go for aerobics since it is the most preconceived exercise that women love to get to. This includes climbing, jogging, Pilates classes, and yoga. When you talk about weight lifting to a woman, you might come out as offensive because it is known to be a man's domain. This has led to the avoidance of weightlifting by women around the world. It has been recorded that approximately 10% of women who are at the age of 45, train with weights, in 2014, when millions of women went to the gym, less than a third considered even picking up the lightest dumbbell.

Women are not aware how strength training can improve their endurance, bone density, improve their performance on daily activities or reduce their body fat.

If women could only get into weight training, they would reap benefits that are beyond their wildest imagination. According to studies done by Harvard, it has been shown that aerobic exercises are way below strength training. Weight training also known as resistance training, offers benefits like:

- Protection against diabetes, arthritis, obesity, and osteoporosis.
- It increases flexibility and body balance.
- Lowers the blood pressure levels

- Encourages youthful appearance
- Improves the brain or cognitive function
- Boosts confidence

If resistance training is a package full of enormous benefits, why are women not jumping on the bandwagon? In the western world, women's body awareness has been subjected to beautification compared to physical strength. These beliefs have made women focus more on their femininity and beauty, ignoring the muscle building and strength development. A woman's fear comes in when they think that lifting weights will make them look muscular and appear bulk in physique. The fear that is held is not based on anything, because, studies have indicated that women are not wired to grow muscles as men do. Men have testosterone that is the main catalyst of muscle growth.

When women lift weights, they can gain muscle size and shape, but you can't compare to that of a man. To add to the fear that exists in women, when a woman sees a weight training equipment, they normally have an invisible label that is written, "Men Only." Women are not familiar with this commercial equipment, and they feel that, when they are seen unable to use the equipment, they will be ridiculed by the public.

Women need to embrace the fact that weight training takes time when it is done properly. One needs to concentrate when lifting weights; if women can become focused and physical when exercising, they can reap enormous benefits at the gym. The benefits are not only for the body, but it goes deep down into the mind.

Is it possible for a woman to become smarter or help in improving her cognitive capability as time goes by? Some say that the brain function is changeable with resistance training. One interesting benefit of weight training revolves around intelligence. Aging is a universal cause of cognitive decline. Studies that have been carried out in the recent decade show that weight training can decrease the brain shrinkage which is as a result of aging. More so, it increases the neuron creation and growth in women who are below the age of 30 and helps them get access to their full cognitive capacity. It was indicated in one of these studies, that women who had mild cognitive impairment, were referred to a gym, for a six-month weight training program to counter the malady.

The outcome of this study indicated that women had improved their memory and functioning of their conflict resolution mechanism. It was reported by Professor Teresa Liu-Ambrose, that the results indicated an improvement of brain function and cognitive performance when strength training was suggested.

Weightlifting is a focus demanding activity because lifting weights require a decent amount of effort, this by itself, improves the brain function. The brain grows as a response to the weight training and as the lifestyle of an individual becomes sedentary, the brain capability deteriorates.

For older women, engaging in weight training at home using dumbbells and hand weights, can be a simple yet inexpensive way to improve their quality of life and health.

Lifting weights enable the aged woman to benefit from an improvement of cardiovascular health, like low-risk arthritis, diabetes, low blood pressure, insomnia, depression, and even the negative effect that menopause can cause. Additionally, it can help to prevent osteoporosis, hip pain, knee pain, and it will also improve their balance.

Aging women do not need to surrender to frailing weak bodies anymore. Weight training can improve muscle strength and bone strength in women of all ages. Looking at women who are at the age of between 47 and 55 years, they tend to undergo menopausally. This is linked to both psychological and physical problem. The changes on the physical side are caused by the slowdown of estrogen hormones. These changes can cause the body fat to increase which risks diabetes and heart disease. There is also the loss of muscles. This means that women will become weaker and they will tend to develop issues related to osteoporosis.

It has been proved by studies, that women who strength train on a regular basis, can improve their bone density and reduce the loss of bone mass. These women between the age of 50 and 70 improved their strength in physical activities, muscle improvement, and enjoyed a better lifestyle. Women have a very bad notion when it comes to weightlifting, what they don't know is that they are the biggest beneficiaries of strength training than anyone else.

After a research which had been taken by Harvard in nursing homes, it was indicated that muscle strength in women improved by over 113% over a period of 10 weeks, after weightlifting. Other residents were able to walk with canes, from walkers. Women can remain independent in their 80's if they have been weightlifting. This will increase their happiness and improve their lives. It is never too late to start lifting weights, regardless of the person's age.

Women have experienced a stereotype when it comes to weightlifting, and it has started being shaken. There has been the constant definition of a modern woman as slim, weak, and small. Beauty is now being defined as the healthy and strong women. No other forms of exercise can come next to strength training. The Director of fitness research at Quincy, explained how women lose approximately 5 pounds of muscle mass every ten years after they hit menopause. The number doubles and the rate of metabolism slow by a rate of 3% every decade. This leads to increased weight and reduced activity. This normally raises the heart diseases, cancer, diabetes, and other forms of diseases. Strength training can regain the loss of these muscles in a matter of weeks.

The benefit of resistance training is a lot, those who train regularly can significantly improve the following areas:

- Improved cardiovascular health
- Stronger bone structure
- Cancer
- Low risk of arthritis development
- Boost self-esteem
- Improved mental focus
- Better flexibility and balance

- Overall body and health wellness.

Women can still tap into the strength and vitality they possessed in their youth when they lift weights. The good part is that in many situations, they will be stronger than anyone can believe.

Chapter 2: The Mindset Around Strength Training

The mindset and exercises seem to be very common topics in the United States of America. You will come across several facts about the relationship between body esteem and exercise. Among the most common are:

- Below 30% of people meet the recommended amounts of exercises that our body needs. People between 18 years and 24 years are the most likely people who like engaging in exercises.
- It is recommended that about 30 mins a day should be spent on exercises for a normal adult. This is with the aim of maintaining a healthy weight.
- When it comes to women, above 85% of them, wish or want to lose weight. When you look at men, below 30 % of them, have complained about their body weight.
- Over half of the women who are aged between 18 years and 24 years prefer to be hit by lightning compared to being fat, but again, two-thirds of them prefer to lazy around and do nothing and be dumb compared to being fat.

These are some facts that complement what is happening in our society today. On the other side, women are getting a lot of pressure from the media for them to get thin and toned. We have seen this in many shows that are geared to getting fat women into shape in a matter of weeks. We have also seen how other female gym instructors broadcast their sessions live, showing women how they can get their bodies into shape. Apart from these, some people are selling products that preach to women that they can get into shape in a matter of weeks, it has become a business that is being sold to women, and they are getting into all manner of programs.

We have also seen how it has been in the media on how the US is an obese nation, and the word about exercises is the salvation of women who don't want to get obese. When you combine these messages, you get a very dangerous cocktail, making women to go to extra miles to be fit and get the bodies they want no matter the cost.

The thinking and reasoning about strength exercises

There are a variety of reasons as to why women exercise, it might be to regain shape after pregnancy, it might be due to the influence they have been induced to by their friends, family, and life partners, or it might be a genuine weight loss desire. On the more long-term side, some want to gain muscle and even strength.

Women who exercise are on the verge of creating very healthy bodies and prevent chronic diseases like heart disease and diabetes. Additionally, women also can exercise to increase their mood and even improve their memory. In a research conducted in 2003 by Fairburn, Shafran, and Cooper, they found that exercise was linked to the reduction of stress, improve the quality of sleep, and even increase the body's energy.

There are two esteems that are affected by exercises; this is body esteem and self-esteem. When we look at self-esteem, we are talking about a stable form of worthiness or personal worth. There has been a ton of research that has attempted to show the relationship between self-esteem and exercises. In 2010, a team of scientists discovered that there is very little significance in the difference between self-esteem on people who exercise and those who don't exercise. What was more significant was the differences in body esteem, especially in women.

Now, what is the difference between body esteem and self-esteem? When we talk about body esteem, we are closely talking about body image. It seems similar to self-esteem, but it's majorly related to how a lady feels about her body and how she takes care of it. When we talk about body esteem, we are looking at a woman's opinion of how attractive she is, and how beautiful her body is.

There is an important aspect of body esteem that we should point out, and this is the social comparison theory. Social comparison theory looks at how people use social standard, financial progress, and other to evaluate themselves against the rest of the people around them; this is because most opinions, abilities, and attitudes are not easily verified other than in the social perspective.

Having said all the above, let us now put it all into perspective on strength training.

Strength training is also referred to as resistance training. It is the ability to grow your muscles for them to perform work more efficiently. Strength training is achieved when the muscle contracts and expands against variable and constant resistance to increase muscle tone and strength. It has been recommended by the American Sports Medicine that women should include strength training in their regular exercise routines. When regular strength training is included in the training program, it has shown that joints and ligaments' structure and functions improve incredibly well. It is the best remedy for back pain, it provides endurance, and increases the strength of the muscles.

Women who are dedicated to cutting weight loss normally go through a fat loss program that is intense, depending on their goals. Once this level is achieved, there is need to maintain the body achieved after the fat loss; here is where strength training comes in. It is what will help a lady maintain a fat-free body mass. To make it even better, when a woman is working out to reduce weight, if there is a combination of strength training and cardiovascular training, there is a high chance of increasing the weight loss target and maintain a good weight.

How often, how much, and how hard should one train?

There should be several variations of aerobic exercises. You can do a bike ride and on the next day, switch it up to walking. This reduces the boredom of exercising on one routine. The best way one can do it is by ensuring that you select an exercise that you can frequently do, and it is enjoyable. It is not good to skip consecutive days without working out because our benefits of training will be lost easily.

It is recommended that you do strength training exercises regularly, to achieve the greatest results for women. One must engage in aerobic exercises more than four times in a week and also engage in strength exercises, about two to three times in a week. It is not simple to get into this framework of training in the first week because your mindset is not in tune with this kind of program. But start out by working out between 30 mins to an hour. According to experts, it is best to split your exercise into shorter yet frequent training periods. This helps to avoid having an excuse, for not having enough time to exercise.

How will I know that I am working hard enough?

There is a simple way of measuring your intensity, and it is called a Talk Test Method. This is how it works, if you are an active lady who enjoys an intense light workout and you are active, you can do something else while doing your exercise like singing. Holding a conversation when you are doing moderate or medium intense workout with your partner or trainer should be easy. An activity is at this moment considered vigorous when the lady becomes too winded, and she is not capable of having a conversation with you when doing the exercise.

Perceived exertion

You can also rate your exercise intensity by the effect it has on your body while doing your exercise is what perceived exertion is. You should always work with the intention of performing at a moderate or hard level. When you improve your fitness level, you will be in a better position of performing at a faster rate while you are still at a moderate perceived exertion.

Perceived exertion scale

You can also use the scale below to guide you in determining how intense your exercises are. As a lady who is starting out on the journey of exercising, it is best you begin at, at the most, a three perceived perception and move slowly up to 3 then a 6 and carry onwards. The most favorable level you can perform your exercises at is a 5 or 6; this will be very effective if you want to lose weight.

1 No effort applied
2 Extremely simple and light
3 A slight light
4 Light
5 Medium rate
6 Difficult
7 Hard
8 Intense
9 Maximum effort about to be used
10 Extreme effort used; cannot work further

Heart Rate

In medium/moderate exercise, the heart rate of a lady is at maximum, should approximately be at 60% to 70%, though it solely depends on the age of the lady.

Estimations of a woman's heart rate, you should subtract the age of the person from 220, an example is, a lady aged 50, her heart rate is calculated easily by 220-50=170 beats per minute. Now, with our percentages above, it should look as follows:

60 percent: 170 x 0.60 = 102 bpm

70 percent: 170 x 0.70=119 bpm

Therefore, if a 50-year-old lady is involved in a moderate workout routine, her heart rate is between 102 and 119 bpm in any activity.

For a lady who is into vigorous activity should aim for a heart rate of between 70 and 90 & of her max heart rate. Follow the formula we have looked into and substitute the percentages.

For instance, if a 35-year-old lady looks to calculate her heart rate, it should be as follows:

220-35=185 bpm.

70 percent: 185 x 0.70=129.5bpm

90 percent: 185 x 0.90=166.5bpm

Therefore, a heart rate that is at 130 and 166.5 bpm will need to be maintained by a 35-year-old woman while under intense workout.

Chapter 3: Equipment Needed For Strength Training

Numerous pieces of equipment 's needed to get your strength-training regime started. That's why joining a gym initially should be considered. Unfortunately, some of the equipment you require to carry out your strength training workout is quite expensive. The cost of membership to a gym will allow you access to all of this equipment. Then over time if you wish to continue your workouts at home you can save money to buy the equipment you need.

1. Weight Machine

This machine uses gravity as its primary source of resistance and will help over time to increase muscle mass. There are several different forms of weight machines you can use as part of your strength-training workout.

Type 1: Stack Machine

Also referred to as a Rack Machine, it comes with a set of large rectangular plates that's been pierced by a vertical bar. You choose your desired weight by inserting pins into the weight. Any plates that sit below where the pin has been inserted will not rise as you carry out a particular exercise.

The great thing about using such a machine is it provides you with several different levels of resistance over a range of motions. However, although some adjustments need to be made for you to lift these weights, you will find the adjustments that need to be made are very small.

How the bars are lifted will vary from one machine to another. Some of these machines are fitted with a roller at the top of the bar that then sits on a lever. When this lever is raised the bar is then able to go up, and the roller moves along the lever so making sure the bar remains vertical.

There are other machines where the bar is attached to a hinge on a lever, and this causes the swaying of the bar and plates as the lever moves up and down. On other stack machines, the bars are attached to a cable or belt, which will run through a pulley or over a wheel. The other end of this cable will then be attached to either a handle or a strap that you need to hold onto or wrap around your body. Again this strap or handle is attached to the lever, and once you begin pulling on it, it'll cause the bars to lift.

Normally you'll notice each bar on the machine is marked with a number. Generally what you find on most machines is the number that's marked on the machine is either for the weight of the plate itself or to tell you what the combined weight of the bars above it is. There are some machines, which use a number that'll give you the force at which when used that actuation point of the machine is achieved. However, on some machines the number that appears on the plates simply is an index counting the number of plates being lifted by you.

Some of the earlier stack machines available, which are known as "Nautilus," were a combination of both lever and cables. Plus they also came with some additional elements to them such as a chinning bar.

Type 2: Plate Loaded Machine

This type of machine uses standard barbell plates rather than captive stacks of plates. It's made up of a bar end on to which the plates are hung using many simple machines to then convey the force of it to the person using it.

Machines designed for strength training will have a very high mechanical advantage over other types as they need to make room for a large number of plates over a large range of movements which allows them to follow a path and converge at one end or the other.

What you'll find with these machines is the motion tends not to be vertical, and the net resistance is often equal to the cosine of the angle about the movement to the vertical.

For example, an incline press machine has a single lever, which comes with the plates halfway up from the handles to the fulcrum. When used you'll notice that the plates then move at a 45-degree angle from the vertical, which then causes the lever to provide a leverage advantage of 2:1.

Whereas when it comes to a bent over rowing machine, this has been designed to ensure your grip is between the plate and the fulcrum. In turn, this helps to amplify the force you need to apply on the lever to lift the weights.

2. Resistance Bands

Most people are unsure as to what resistance bands do and how they need to be used. But you may find these effects as they provide you with a great way to workout when away from home or unable to get to the gym. They can certainly add a bit of variety to your strength-training workout.

If you intend to use resistance bands be aware, there are certain problems you may face.

Problem 1 – You may find the resistance feels different. This is because when you use free weights, it's gravity that decides where the weight is coming from. So what you find is that it offers more resistance during one part of the movement than another.

However when you use resistance bands the tension on them is constant which makes it feel like you're working a lot harder. They work in much the same way as a cable weight machine does allow you to keep constant tension on your muscles.

You'll also find you're using more of the stabilizer muscles in your body to make sure the band remains properly aligned as you perform each exercise, so this, in turn, adds a completely different dynamic to each move you perform.

Problem 2 – You may not find resistance bands as challenging as when you're carrying out exercises using dumbbells or machines. With weights, you will, of course, know just how much you're lifting, whereas with the bands you can only go by how it feels and how much tension is on them. However, this doesn't mean your workout won't be as good.

To make sure your muscles don't notice any difference between using resistance bands or weights you need to make sure you're using the right form when exercising. Plus you must make sure you're placing the right level of tension on the bands.

One big advantage to be gained from using resistance bands rather than weights is, of course, they allow you to create resistance from various directions. Not only can you create resistance from in front, but to the side, overhead and below.

Problem 3 – The biggest problem you'll face when using resistance bands for the first time, is to know how to use them correctly. Yes, it will be a little confusing at first, but one thing to keep in mind is you're able to perform the same exercises with these bands as you would with free weights, the only difference relates to where the bands are positioned.

So Why Give Resistance Bands A Go?

- Unlike free weights, using resistance bands allows you to perform various exercises in a variety of different ways. Not only will this help to change the way the exercise feels, as it's being carried out, but also helps to change the way in which your body's being exercised.

- Of all the equipment you can purchase for your strength training program, this is one of the least expensive. Resistance bands cost somewhere between $6 and $20 depending on where you buy them from and whom they're made the buy.

- Not only is this type of equipment suitable for people who have been working out for some time, but they are also effective for those who have only just begun to work out.

3. Exercise Ball

The main advantage to doing exercises with an exercise ball is it allows you to perform a wide range of exercises. Also known as a Swiss ball, this particular piece of equipment, like the resistance band, is very cheap to buy and comes in a variety of different sizes. So finding one that not only suits your budget but also your requirements shouldn't prove a problem.

Most exercise balls you purchase are constructed from soft elastic and will measure between 35 and 85 centimeters (14 to 34 inches) in diameter. They are filled with air, and you have the opportunity to change the amount of air within them by either putting more air in or by letting some out. Although it's used for physical therapy exercises or athletic training, you'll find the exercise ball a very useful piece of equipment.

4. Dumbbells

This, of course, is one of the most common pieces of equipment that you should be using as part of your strength-training program. You can either use these separately or in pairs.

Although the dumbbell has been around for hundreds of years the shape of dumbbells we use today didn't come into being until the early 17th Century. Today there are three forms of dumbbells that you should be using as part of your strength training for beginners program. These are:

Type 1: Adjustable Dumbbells

This particular type of dumbbell consists of a metal part where the middle part is often etched with a crosshatch (knurling) pattern so that gripping it is a lot easier. You can add or remove weight plates (disks) from this by sliding them onto the bar through the holes and then securing them in place with either a collar or a clip. However there are some adjustable dumbbells that to keep the plates in place require a large nut to be screwed into position, this type of dumbbell is known as a "spinlock" model.

Today most of the dumbbells sold commercially come with sophisticated and easy to use weight increment adjustments.

Type 2: Fixed-Weight Dumbbells

These require a lot less to buy than the adjustable dumbbells but are similar in shape to them. Often these are made from cast iron and then coated with either rubber or neoprene to make holding them a lot easier and a lot more comfortable. However, these cost considerably more than those, which happens to be made up of a rigid plastic shell into which concrete has then been poured.

Type 3: Selectorized Dumbbells

These types of dumbbells come with many different weighted plates that you're able to change easily while they are placed on the stand. This is done by turning a dial or moving the pin to a new position to choose the weight you wish to lift, instead of having to add or remove plates from the bar manually.

The great thing about using these dumbbells is when you need to change the weight according to various exercises you are doing, it can be done a lot more easily and quickly. Of course, such dumbbells take up considerably less room than the conventionally adjustable dumbbells as you don't have to worry about storing different weight plates.

5. Barbell

If you're going to be using this type of equipment as part of your strength training program, you should opt for the much shorter and lighter ones initially. Then when you feel your strength improving you should use much larger and heavier ones.

Barbells are available measuring from 1.2m (4 feet) to 2.4 (8 feet) in length. However, the bars that measure more than 7.2feet (2.2 merest) are the kind normally used by powerlifters and can be difficult to find. In fact, the only place where you may find such barbells is your local gym.

The actual central part of this equipment does vary somewhat. Some are just 25mm (0.98 inches) in diameter, while others can measure up to 51mm (2 inches) in diameter. Just as with dumbbells and the bars used on weight machines, have a crosshatch (knurled) pattern etched onto them, as it helps to make gripping them a lot easier. However, if you'd like a better grip or more comfort, then you need to think about investing in some weight lifting gloves. These look just like any other gloves but come with the ends of the fingers cut off and include some material on the palm part to make gripping the bars a lot easier.

Just like some forms of dumbbells, this equipment is designed to allow you to put different weights on the bar. The weights can be slid onto the bar and held in place with either a collar or clip.

Again you need to be aware there are various forms of barbells you can use to help improve your muscle mass and strength.

Type 1: Standard Barbell

Although they carry the same name, the standard barbells tend to have very little in common except of course for how wide they are. There are in fact two things that these barbells share. The first being the loading area tends to be much thinner compared to what you'd find on barbells used for weightlifting in competitions. Most of the standard barbells have a diameter of between 25mm (1 inch) and 28mm (1.1 inches). They also tend to be threaded or plain and so will require a different sort of collar or clip to keep the weights in place.

The second thing these types of barbells have in common is they are often made from one single solid piece of metal.

Type 2: EZ Curl Barbell

This is a variant of the standard barbell that's mainly used when doing bicep curls, upright rows or lying triceps extensions. The profile of the bar in the area you grip is curved, and as a result, when using it, it allows your wrists and forearms to take a much more neutral position. As a result of this, the risk of you causing a repetitive strain injury in these areas of your body are greatly reduced.

You need to be aware when using the EZ curl barbell, that when carrying out the bicep curl exercise it will prevent you from contracting the bicep muscles completely. The only way you can contract your biceps fully is through ensuring your wrist is fully supinated. So you may find using this piece of equipment to carry out this particular exercise is not as effective as you would have hoped.

Type 3: Fixed Barbell

These are the kind you'll find most often at your local gym, and the bar itself is usually fairly short which has weights already attached to the bar and have been welded in place. You'll often find with this sort of barbell, the plates (weights) themselves have been covered in either plastic or rubber.

Typically the fixed barbells you use in a gym will carry weights of between 5 and 40 kg on them. These types of barbells are much handier to have as they take up considerably less space than the other types. Not only are they shorter in length than the other but also, you don't have to concern yourself with having additional plates to store away.

The fixed barbell is much more useful to have as it allows you to perform a variety of different exercises where the use of very little weight is needed. Plus you'll find they provide you with the perfect starting point for strength training before you think about moving on to using other types of barbells mentioned above. Also, you'll find these allow for a much speedier transition between using various weights if you're performing various exercises that need to use multiple weights in quick succession.

Type 4: Thick Handed Barbell

This is a more of a specialist item and is designed in such a way to help challenge your grip when lifting the bar with weights on it. This type of barbell is the kind that's used by those participating in competitions when deadlifts and overhead presses need to be performed.

Type 5: Triceps Barbell

This particular barbell functions in much the same way as the EZ curl barbell does. The triceps barbell is made up of two parallel handles that have been mounted in a cage. You will use this particular piece of equipment to perform triceps extensions as well as hammer curls.

Type 6: Trap Barbell

The trap barbell is a diamond shaped bar in the middle, which requires you to stand and grasp the bar by its handles with a neutral grip. The way in which this barbell is used ensures the center of gravity is much closer to you as you lift. Primarily this sort of bar will be used to carry out deadlifts and shrugs.

6. Adjustable Weight Bench

This is the perfect piece of equipment to have to perform chest and back exercises on. Plus it's also perfect for carrying out a quick abdominal workout or a few triceps dips. Along with adjustable weight benches, you'll find there are some flat ones as well. However, the adjustable type is best as it allows you to raise and lower the bench when carrying out exercises, which helps, in turn, to make them much more challenging.

7. Exercise Mat

The final thing you'll need to carry out your exercises is an exercise mat. This is great for doing your abdominal workouts on as well as many toning exercises.

Chapter 4: Strength Training Workout for Women

This strength workout has been specifically designed for women regardless of age, which means that you can follow it no matter if you are in your early twenties or a senior who is approaching your sixties.

There is nothing advanced about it, and even if you are a total beginner, you should be able to jump into it and start performing the exercises. Although some of the exercises are performed with different weights, you should know that this is optional.

For the exercises that require barbells, she uses a rolled carpet while having two bags of equal weight filled with anything she can find hanging at the sides of the carpet.

As you realize, you don't need any equipment instead of by using your imagination; you can easily use stuff that can be found almost anywhere for your workout.

You can no longer use as an excuse for not working on your strength the fact that you don't have the right equipment. Instead, take what you can find and start working out without searching for any excuses s not to do it.

With that said, let's dig into the strength workout that will transform your body once and for all and give you that leaner, well-shaped and more sculpted body you've always wanted to have...

Warm up Routine

Warm up is what makes your body ready for the workout, and it should not be skipped under any circumstances. This is where you prepare for the workout, and it tells your body to get ready for what's coming. Some of the benefits you'll get from warming up include the following:

- Highly limiting the risk of getting injured when performing the exercises.
- Increases oxygen flow to your muscles and decreases the lactic acid.
- Makes your body better at burning more calories per workout.
- Easier to gain muscle control thus allowing you to perform the exercises easier.
- Preventing your body from fatigue while decreasing the workout pain.

Unfortunately, my experience is that women don't realize how important it is to warm up properly until something bad happens. My wife used to be in the group of women who didn't care about warming up.

I don't know how many times I told her that it was crucial for her to warm up, but she just waved away my arguments and said that nothing had happened to her so far and she would not waste her time on it.

However, this was about to change soon because during one of the strength workouts at our apartment, she strained her thigh muscle while she was doing an exercise and suddenly she could barely walk properly without having pain.

This kept bothering her for several weeks, but once she healed, she continued with the same behavior, which was to start performing the exercises directly without paying attention to warming up.

Not long after she recovered from the first injury, she injured the same thigh a second time and again she was forced to walk around with pain for several weeks while handling with the frustration of not being able to exercise.

I told her that if she stopped being so stubborn and started listening to my advice on warming up, she would not need to worry about getting injured. If she at least spends 5 minutes warming up, she would not need to worry about getting injured again.

Fortunately, she listened to my advice, and since that day, she never had any problems with injuries again. Today, she thankfully praises me in front of other women who refuse to warm up and tells them about the consequences.

My point with this story is to make you understand that warming up is vital to keeping you safe from injuries while allowing you to get the maximum from your workouts. Remember, in the end, it is solely your responsibility to warm up properly, as no one will do the work for you!

All of those warming up exercises are pretty much mobile which means that they can be performed at any time at any place with minimum space, which gives you great opportunities to work on your strength no matter where in the world you are.

Spot Jogging

The best thing about this way of warming up is that you barely need space to perform it. To perform it, you just simulate jogging, the same way like if you were jogging outside- but without moving forward (unless you live in a castle)!

My wife always uses this as a part of her overall warm-up routine, and she says that it helps her to get the blood pumping and have to get her body ready for the upcoming exercise.

Duration: 120 seconds

Quick Feet

In this warm-up exercise, you should run in place with your weight on your toes. Try to keep the speed at about 70% of your maximum workout pace to increase your heart rate and get the blood flowing in your veins.

Just like spot jogging, this warm-up exercise requires minimum space, and you can perform it almost anywhere.

Duration: 60 seconds

High Knees

Stand in place while having your arms stretched in front of you. Start then to lift up your knees –one at a time, so that they are touching the palms of your hands. Perform this exercise at about 70% of your maximum speed.

Duration: 60 seconds

Butt Kickers

Start by slight jogging on the spot while kicking you're out with the heels of your feet. Use your arms just as if you were running, which means that you are holding them close to your body while moving them back and forward.

It's worth emphasizing that you should do this in a smooth motion without forcing the heel too much. You need to remember this is a warm-up and not an exercise where you should perform at your maximum.

Duration: 60 seconds

Lower Body Exercises
Having a strong lower body allows you to have fabulous and well-formed legs while helping you with daily activities like walking. In this part of the strength workout we will focus mainly on the exercises that are targeting the muscles in your legs, which will help you achieve amazing looking legs- so let's dig into it!

Split Squat
Although my wife hates to perform this exercise, I still consider it as being one of the most powerful for strengthening your legs. It is also great because by performing it you indirectly involve the hamstrings and your back.

Equipment: A pair of dumbbells with equal weights.

Preparation: Grasp and lift up the dumbbells to hip level with a steady grip.

Instructions:

- Take the starting position by standing with feet shoulder-width apart.
- Step forward with an extended step that is about twice your normal walking step.
- Slightly lower your body while focusing the weight on your front leg.
- As you touch the ground with the knee push upwards slowly but avoid stepping back.
- Perform 10-12 repetitions, switch the leg and repeat.

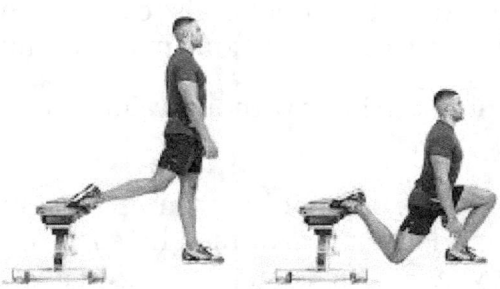

Tip: Try looking slightly at the sky to keep your upper body straight.

Variation: You may vary this exercise by having your back leg propped on a low object.

Precaution: If you are new to the world of strength training start to perform the exercise without weights to learn the basic range of motion.

Single Leg Deadlift
This exercise will do wonders for your hamstrings and glutes! It is also by far one of the most popular exercises for improving your strength which qualifies it as an important part of your workout.

Equipment: A pair of dumbbells with equal weight.

Preparation: Grasp and lift up the dumbbells at hip level with a steady grip.

Instructions:

- Begin with feet shoulder width apart, while keeping your back straight.
- Lift the back leg a few inches off the ground and keep it hovering.
- Inhale while slightly lowering your upper body, constantly keeping your back straight.
- Exhale while lifting yourself upwards, keeping the weight focused on the front leg.

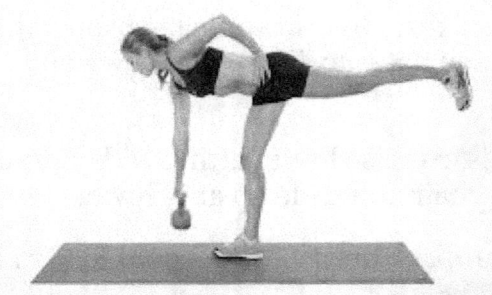

Tip: Try looking slightly at the sky to keep your upper body flat easier.

Variation: An easy way to vary the single deadlift is to switch the legs after every repetition, instead of performing 10-12 repetitions in a row and then switching.

Precaution: Ensure proper form and start without weights if you are new to the exercise.

Traditional Squat
If you have ever participated in the popular body pump session, you know how painful this exercise is, and in my experience most women hate it! However, it works, and it will give you great shaped legs if you just focus on performing it with enough focus and determination.

Equipment: Barbell with equal weights at each side.

Preparation: Make sure to position the barbell slightly below the level of your shoulders.

Instructions:

- Tighten your abdominal muscles and grasp the barbell with a steady grip.
- Inhale while lowering yourself slowly until you are in a chair sitting position.
- Exhale while slowly raising yourself while keeping your back straight.

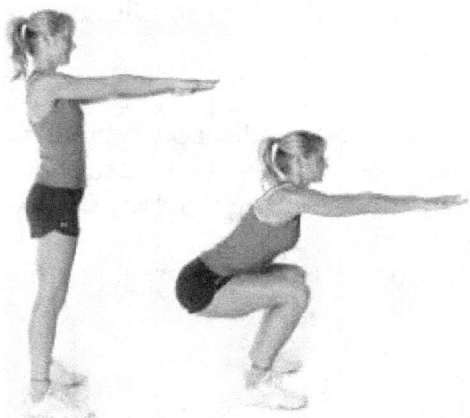

Tip: Add an object not higher than your lower leg, perform the squat and as soon as you touch the object, raise yourself back up. This will allow you to improve your balance and perform the exercise better.

Variation: You may vary this exercise by squatting with your back against a wall, just like if you were sitting on a chair and slide up and down.

Precaution: Don't curve your back inwards as it could lead to injuries in your back.

Abdominals and Core
I know you want to get sculpted and strong abs in the shortest time possible, but I must disappoint you and say that it will usually take you a while to get rid of the fat on your

belly. You must realize that you can't burn fat in one specific spot. Instead, your body decides when it's time to get rid of the belly fat.

What you can do is just to keep working on your strength and follow a healthy diet where you avoid junk food and other tasty temptations like cakes, soda, candy, etc. I ensure you that if you do so, your body is going to reward you by burning the belly fat and give you those sculpted abs!

Now, I have researched the abdominal and core exercises for women and found that those listed below are the most efficient ones for sculpturing your abs and strengthening your core, so let's dig into it!

Plank Exercise
My research shows that this is the ultimate exercise for increasing the strength of your oblique's, which are located on either side of your abdominals. These are a pain and don't be fooled by the simplicity because they will do wonders for your core strength.

Equipment: Nothing specific, but a cushion for the elbows is recommended.

Preparation: Kneel down while keeping the arms extended (do not lock elbows) in front of you.

Instructions:

- Raise your upper body with your underarms while raising the legs by pushing up on your toes.
- Inhale while keeping your body completely extended and hover above the ground for 15-30 seconds.
- Exhale while releasing your body slowly to the ground.
- Rest for 30 seconds and then repeat.

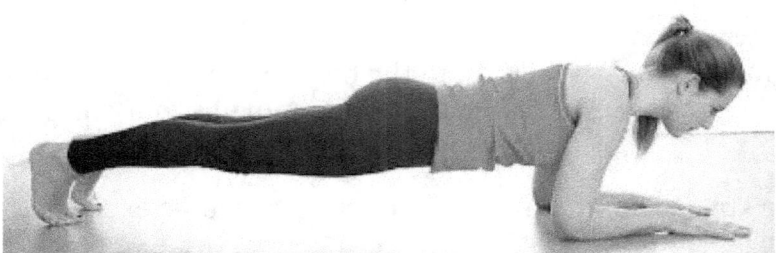

Tip: You may perform the exercise in front of a mirror to ensure proper form.

Variation: You may vary this exercise by raising one of your arms in front of you while keeping your position for 15 seconds and then repeat with your other arm.

Precaution: Make sure to breathe normally during the whole exercise.

Bicycle Exercise
This is a great exercise for improving the overall strength of your abdominal muscles, so it's an obvious part of the workout in this book.

Equipment: Nothing specific, but a mat for your back is recommended.

Preparation: Lie down on the ground.

Instructions:

- Grasp the back of your head slightly with your hands.
- Exhale while moving the right elbow across your body and touch the left knee with it.
- Inhale while lowering yourself to the starting position.
- Repeat with the other elbow.

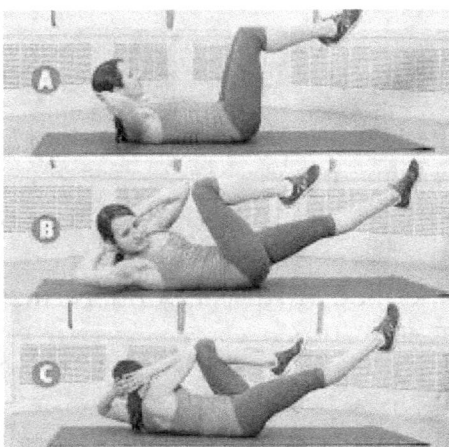

Tip: I recommend that you use a mat, as it will make the exercise more comfortable for your back.

Variation: An easy way to add variation to the bicycle exercise is to attach your foot to the ground and have your legs forming an A while moving your elbows across the body in the same way.

Precaution: Make sure to breathe normally during the whole exercise.

Reverse Crunch
Reverse crunches are highly effective for improving the lower abdominals, and they have been around since the very beginning of strength training.

Equipment: Placing a mat with you to provide comfort for your back is recommended.

Preparation: lay down on the ground.

Instructions:

- Lie down and grip an object to hold onto (e.g., a dumbbell).
- Exhale while lifting your hips off the ground and moving your knees toward your face.
- Inhale while extending your legs without allowing them to touch the ground.

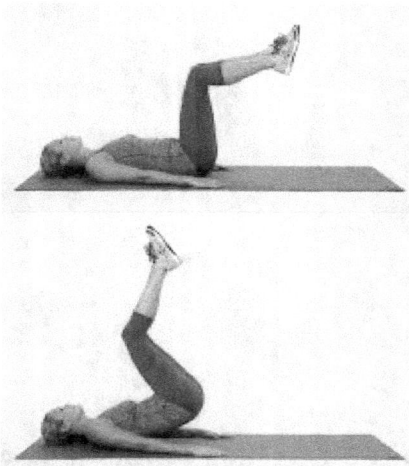

Tip: Focus on keeping your abs contracted during each repetition.

Variation: You can vary the reverse crunch by lying down and grasping the back of a small bench while having your feet hovering above the ground as the starting position.

Precaution: Make sure to breathe normally during the whole exercise.

Upper Body Exercises

This section of the workout is designed to improve the strength of your upper body, which includes your arms, shoulders, and back. Some of the benefits of having a stronger body include improved metabolism and decreased risk of osteoporosis.

Plus, a stronger upper body will also allow you to perform other activities easier, such as carrying groceries, lifting your children and taking care of the daily household without constantly feeling pain in your body.

In other words, by working on your upper body, you have nothing to lose but everything to gain. With that said, let's dig into the exercises!

Bent Knee Push Up

This exercise is a light version of the standard push-up, but it doesn't mean that it's not efficient.

Equipment: Place a mat under your knees to provide more comfort.

Preparation: Kneel down on the floor while keeping your upper body straight.

Instructions:

- Lift your knees up so that they are forming the letter 'L.'
- Exhale while lowering your body down and contracting your abs.
- Inhale while lifting yourself up to the starting position without locking your elbows.

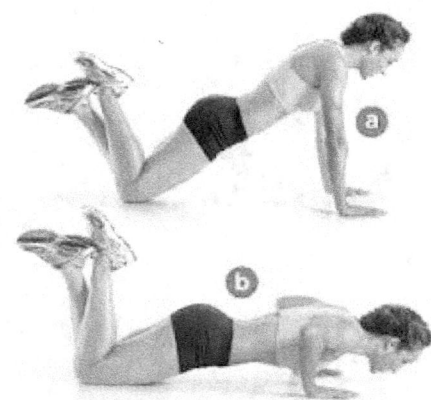

Tip: Use something soft to provide a cushion to your knees and to make the exercise more comfortable.

Variation: Once you feel stronger in your body you should try switching to the standard pushups which are more demanding but more efficient.

Precaution: It is vital to breathe normally during the whole exercise.

Standing Shoulder Press
If you have been looking for ways to improve the strength of your shoulders, this is the ultimate exercise you should be focusing on. It will also indirectly involve other muscle groups like triceps and traps which is awesome!

Equipment: A pair of dumbbells of equal weight.

Preparation: Lift up the dumbbells just above the shoulders.

Instructions:

- Stand shoulder-width apart while keeping your back straight.
- Exhale by pushing up the dumbbells until your arms are stretched, but don't lock the elbows.
- Inhale by slowly lowering the dumbbells in a controlled manner back to the starting position.

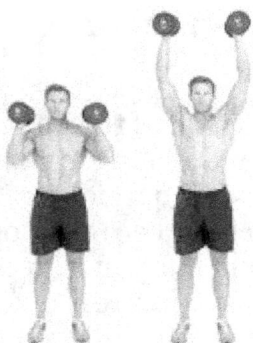

Tip: You may vary this exercise by using a barbell instead of dumbbells.

Variation: You may vary this exercise by sitting on a chair and performing the same routine.

Precaution: It is vital to breathe normally during the whole exercise.

Conclusion

Thank you for making it through to the end of the book, Strength: Strength Training for Women, we hope that it was informative enough to provide you with the necessary information and guidelines to change your outlook as a woman to weight training. After reading this book, we believe that you have become more intentional into going for weight training workouts, and we would like you to get more knowledge on different variations of the exercise. Don't just stop after reading this book; there are tons of nutritional information that you need to accumulate to make your strength training sessions more efficient and effective.

The next stage is to get started in weight training. Subscribe to a gym and seek the guidance of the gym instructor on the schedules we have identified for you. Our trainer might change a few styles, because they are a better place of understanding your body, and you should be flexible enough to take the advice of heart.

Studies have shown that women are even better and way slower when they engage in weight training exercises. Once you have started getting into the rhythm of strength training, you will have a better chance of working more productively, grow better, and increase or reduce weight as per your needs.

Finally, if you found this book informative enough, a review on Amazon is always appreciated!

www.ingramcontent.com/pod-product-compliance
Lightning Source LLC
Chambersburg PA
CBHW081139280526
45787CB00007B/3152

* 9 7 8 1 5 4 9 9 0 8 3 2 3 *